Go To My Blog
AWESOME Ways to Burn Fat and Build Muscle

My wife is a registered dietitian and I'm a fitness nut. Check out my blog for some great fitness tips. Here are my top articles:

- 37 Mind-Blowing Tips to Burn Fat & Build Muscle (w/ pics and links)
- How to Burn Fat & Get Ripped Eating One Meal per Day
- The 39 Coolest Fitness Blogs in the World (plus their most mind-blowing articles)
- 6 "Dirty" Secrets the Fitness Industry Uses to Make Billions (don't fall for these tricks)

Please share these articles on Facebook and Twitter!

And while you're there, don't forget to sign up to my email newsletter where I share free tips, updates, and exclusive articles. I'll even give you a copy of my free report "The ULTIMATE Muscle-Building Dessert"

Get access to all of this at my blog:

www.TheScienceofGettingRipped.com

Can I Ask You a Quick Favor?

If you like this book, I would greatly appreciate if you could leave an honest review on Amazon.

Reviews are very important to us authors, and it only takes a minute to post. At the end of this book please post a review.

Also, please check out my comprehensive manual, "*The Science of Getting Ripped*" for workout plans and tips to burn fat and build muscle.

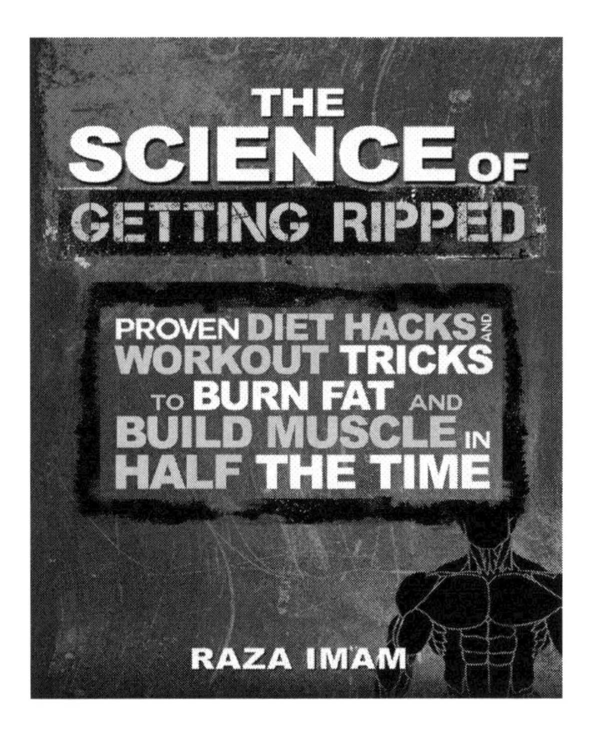

Click here to check it out here:
www.TheScienceofGettingRipped.com

Thank you in advance!

Who This Is For

This is for the average guy who wants to lose fat and build muscle. It's for the busy parent, the entrepreneur, the guy who wants to help others. He needs the physical strength to accomplish his goals, but also the discipline, fortitude, mental toughness, character, and self-respect to handle life's most difficult tasks.

Whether that means turning around a struggling business, volunteering with young kids, or raising a growing family, having a solid physique in addition to the inner strength to blast through life's obstacles and challenges is the key to success.

The ideal reader doesn't want to be a pretty boy fitness model nor a bodybuilder. He reads popular men's health magazines, is interested in technology, and photography, and current events, and sports. He is tech savvy and forward thinking, with aspirations and ambitions for himself and his family. He doesn't want to spend hours a day in the gym. He looks for efficiency and fitness hacks to get him the most results from his workouts.

Here's the thing, most products focus on getting ripped, and this will show you how to do just that. But the way I see it, you don't walk around with your shirt off all day. You DO meet people, solve problems, create plans, help others, encounter obstacles, and live a full life. So why not focus on not only the physical benefits you'll get when you workout, but on the confidence and mental toughness you gain as well? Seems like the best of both worlds to me.

My Story

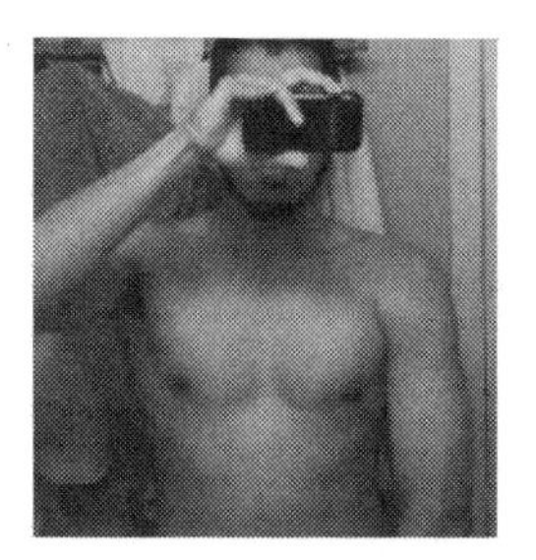 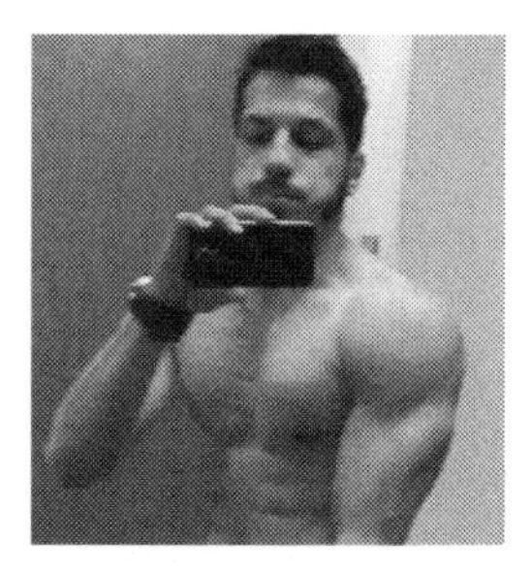

Like most 30-something guys with kids, I have a very busy life. Here's my typical day: An hour-long commute to and from work. Helping my 5 year-old with homework. Giving the kids baths. Putting them to bed. Doing dishes. Hanging out with the wife. And going to bed.

I love working out and used to be heavily involved in martial arts. But I just couldn't keep it up with this crazy schedule. I've been wanting to get back in shape for quite a while, but never had the time to go to the gym consistently. Once I hit 30, I was terrified that I would get the dreaded "skinny fat" body type. You know what I'm talking about. Skinny body with a pot belly.

Now I'm 34 with 3 kids and decided to start writing to help other people get in shape.

Sincerely,

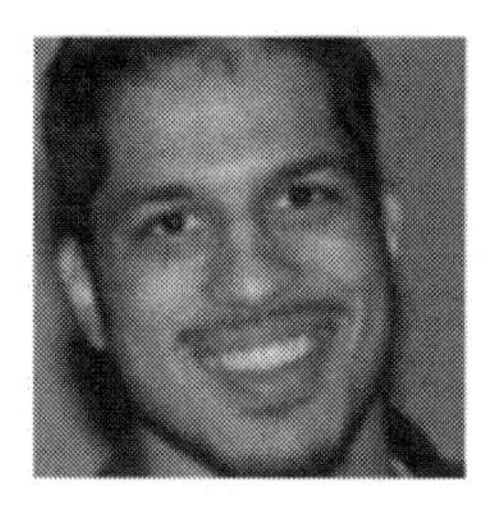

Raza Imam

Table of Contents

Introduction

Losing weight is actually easier than you think. The same goes with building muscle. I know this is kind of hard to believe because there are tons of diet and fitness books out there. They are all based on the assumption that weight loss is difficult and you need THEIR solution to achieve your weight loss goals.

There is also no shortage of health supplements making all sorts of muscle-building claims. In fact, if you really think about it, there is a huge global multi-billion dollar industry built around the promise that people can lose weight and build up muscle so they can finally get the body that they've been dreaming of.

The problem is that most people fail to build up muscle.

They fail to get that sleek physique they desire. The reason for this all-too-predictable failure is easy to understand. You see, if you are going to try to lose weight through dieting, chances are, you will fail. I know that's not pleasant news but that's the reality.

The problem with diets is that while you can lose weight with them, in most cases, the results are not permanent. Even if you were to lose weight, you can still get flabby. I know this seems counter intuitive but this happens all the time. The way most people go about losing weight is they just focus on reducing their weight and don't pay enough attention to making sure they look fit. They lose weight but their bodies don't look all that good. There's nothing sexy about a thin but loose or flabby body!

What is the better alternative?

The better approach to weight loss would be to use exercise to build muscle. When your overall muscle mass goes up, your resting metabolism rate-the rate at which your body burns calories passively-goes up. It takes more energy to maintain your body because of your greater muscle mass. Put simply, you are positioning yourself to burn calories passively instead of having to hit the gym or go on a diet just to cut down on weight.

The higher your resting metabolism, the less effort it takes for you to lose weight. You can eat closer to the amount you're eating now without worrying that you'll be packing on pounds.

The problem with using only exercise

At this point, I know that you're probably all excited about hitting the gym and getting buff. There's a lot to be excited about. Don't get me wrong. But the problem is, if you're just going to use exercise to build your overall muscle mass, you also have to pay attention to the other part of the equation. It's not pretty.

The more you exercise, the more your diet will work against you. Your body will go into starvation mode or otherwise adopt all sorts of "defensive patterns" so you can go back to your "regular" weight.

The best weight loss solution is quite easy on an obvious level: burn the candle from both ends. This means eating fewer calories while eating more muscle-boosting protein and hitting the gym.

Your goal is quite simple: weigh less and look buffed and toned while keeping the weight off permanently. Does this sound too good to be true? Somehow it does but it's also completely doable. This book helps you adopt a lifestyle where you're eating delicious and filling meals while at the same time reducing your calorie intake and boosting muscle mass.

It seems like the best of both worlds. You just have to have to put the right pieces in place.

Chapter 1

Before you begin: mentally program yourself of PERMANENT WEIGHT LOSS SUCCESS

As I mentioned in the introduction, there is a large number of popular diets on the global marketplace. There is no shortage of "latest and greatest" diets that guarantee weight loss. The truth is, these diet books sell precisely due to the fact that they work. I'm going to lie to you. They will help you lose weight here and there.

Your main problem, however, is not losing weight. It is keeping the weight off!

These are two totally different things. Unfortunately, most diet books don't pay enough attention to the number one factor that ensures you persistent weight loss. Again, there are many diets that will produce drastic results. The problem with those diets is that as time goes, the weight comes back. Even worse, you end weighing more than when you started. You end up in a worse place.

What is the missing ingredient? The right mindset!

Before you begin your weight loss regimen and hitting the gym, I need you to adopt the right mindset. Without it, you are going to fail. It really is that simple.

I need you to wrap your mind around the following facts. These are not opinions or advisory material. You have to make these part of your mindset so that you can achieve permanent weight loss. If you fail to believe in any of these, chances are quite high whatever weight loss success you do enjoy will be short-lived. Consider yourself warned!

To achieve, you must first believe

For you to benefit from this book, I need you to believe that all this will work. Without belief, diets simply won't produce persistent benefits. The reason is simple. When you believe something will work for you, it changes your emotional state. You are more curious, motivated and willing to try out things that you haven't done before. When you are in that emotional state, it changes your actions.

Since you're more willing to try things out, you gain the energy to actually get off the fence and turn theory into practice. You actually start to give more careful attention to the meals that you choose to enjoy. You also get the motivation you need to start hitting the gym.

All this flows back to the power of belief. To achieve anything, you must first believe that something will happen. I need you to understand this. If you want this book to deliver solid and real benefits to your life, you must first believe that the things I will tell you will work.

Your mindset impacts your willpower

If you believe that something is worth doing and you have what it takes to do it, you increase your willpower. This is extremely important because any kind of diet involves cutting back on things that are pleasurable.

Let's face it. Eating a large chunk of chocolate cake is more pleasurable than chowing down on a plate of broccoli and chicken breast. Chocolate cake, for most people, wins hands-down all the time. That's the reality that you need to work against. Choosing healthier food requires willpower. You burn through your will power fighting the things that are pleasure but lead to more fat and heavier weight and choosing food that bring less immediate pleasure. Eating less food is not pleasurable but you need to do it.

Without the right mindset, your willpower will be limited and produce fewer effects in your life. Understand this connection between your mindset and your willpower so that you can adopt the right mindset that leads to greater willpower.

Your mindset impacts your self-control and discipline

Getting on a diet takes quite a bit of energy. Unfortunately, things get worse from there. To stay on a diet, you need even more energy. This is where self-control and discipline kick in. You're not the first person to get excited about a hot new diet that has hit the market. Like millions of other people, you buy that diet book off the shelf and can't wait to implement it.
This takes off willpower but you are excited enough to make a hard decision and take action.

What happens next is the most difficult part. You need self-control to stick with your program. Some days are worse than others. There are certain days where you're just tempted to eat as much chocolate cake as you want and cheat on your diet. The more you give in to these temptations, the harder and harder it will be to resist them in the future. Eventually, you just give up. You've been completely thrown off track and stop dieting. The weight comes back and, oftentimes, you end up weighing more than you began.

The secret to all this: having the right mindset. When you understand the connection between your mindset and the amount of self-control and discipline that you have, you are in a better position to avoid temptation. You can adopt mindsets that strengthen your self-control and self-discipline instead of weakening it.

Let me get one thing clear; if you are completely clueless regarding how mindset impacts your self-control and discipline, you're positioning yourself to not have any during times of almost irresistible temptation.

Be aware of your mindset: stop programming yourself for failure

Another key lesson I need you to the internalize is the fact that most people who try diet after diet, program themselves for failure. There are certain thoughts that come to mind that if left unchallenged, will undermine your result.

One, when you make “deals" with yourself where you say, "Well, I'm going to cheat on my diet today. Tomorrow, I'll get back on the wagon." You may be able to get back on the wagon the next day, but compromising now makes you vulnerable to more temptations in the future. Eventually, it becomes harder and harder for you to resist temptation.

Another mindset that you need to guard against, is when you tell yourself, "I'm fat", "I am hopeless", "I will continue to be fat", "I will never get the body that I deserve" or so on and so forth. When you make this quote "I am” statements, you are defining yourself as a failure. You're just telling yourself that this is your identity; that you are designed for failure or that's all you're capable of.

You see, the phrases above are 'defining statements.' You're speaking your identity out to the world. Believe me, your body is paying attention. Your mind might be rationalizing that you're just saying things out of frustration or that you don't or you don't really mean what you're saying. Still, if you're not careful, your body starts living out the reality of your statements. If you say that you're permanently fat or that you are a loser, your body will pick up on this. This reality will be reflected in your eating patterns and in your weight. It is also going to show in your physique.

Be aware of what you're programming yourself to be. If anything, you need to disrupt the process and apply counter programming. Instead, say to yourself "I am... fit, buff, successful or a winner."

Adopt this simple mindfulness technique

The reason why a lot of these mindset facts seems challenging is because most of us have undisciplined minds. This should not be a surprise. People are creatures of pleasure. We tend to want things that feel good now and avoid things that require sacrifice or are outright unpleasant.

While we can intellectually understand that there are certain things that are painful now but bring reward in the future, in practical terms, our bodies put up a fight. We'd rather do something that feels good now. This is how our minds usually work. Unless you take conscious action to retrain your mind, resistance is going to be its default pattern.

One of the most powerful ways to retrain your mind so you can adopt the right weight loss mindset is mindfulness. Whether you use proper meditation techniques, or choose simple mindfulness exercises, you need to adopt some sort of simple mindfulness technique that would enable you to get the right mindset. At the very least, you will be able to boost your willpower. It will also help you recharge your willpower faster.

There are many different mindfulness techniques out there. You can choose visualization, counting your breath, sensing mental images on a moment by moment basis, and so on and so forth. What's important is that you learn a technique for living in the present moment and allowing your mind to relax while, at the same time, strengthening your mental focus. This will enable you to adopt the right mindsets and benefit more from them.

The bottom line

When it comes to the connection between your mindset and your body, you need to change your lifestyle to achieve permanent weight loss. Lifestyle modification requires a ton of willpower. You need to understand this and take action. By simply adopting the mindsets above and practicing a simple mindfulness technique, you build up the inner tools you need for ultimate weight loss and muscle building success.

Chapter 2

Weight loss basics and the power of calorie counting

Weight loss is actually quite simple. In fact, it's almost mathematical. Basic weight loss works in the following way. Your body is always burning calories. By simply reading this book, you're already burning calories. When you walk around and breathe, you burn calories. The act of standing up burns calories. Your body constantly needs energy to pump blood, breathe oxygen, move around, etc.

This energy is measured in terms of calories that come from the food you eat. Pretty simple so far, right? Well, to lose weight, you just need to eat fewer calories than the amount of calories your body already burns. When this happens, you achieve a “net negative” calorie state. Your body starts looking at your stored fat and burns it up for calories. It also looks at the sugar in your blood stream and burns that up for energy.

Another way to achieve a net negative calorie state is to eat the same amount of calories but increase the amount of calories your body burns on both passive and active level. Active calorie burning is when you are doing cardiovascular exercises, working out at the gym or simply walking from point A to point B and going about your business in a typical day. Anything that requires physical energy requires burning calories actively.

Passive calorie burning, on the other hand, is the amount calories your body burns naturally even when you are resting. This is the amount of energy your body needs when you're simply lying down, sleeping or sitting in front of the computer. If you boost the amount of calories your body burns, either passively or actively, you achieve a net negative calorie state.

The third alternative way to burn calories is to simply do both. You simply eat less and increase your physical activity. This is the fastest way to lose weight.

If all this sounds almost too basic, indeed it is. While losing weight follows these rules, there are certain nuances that you need to pay attention to. These small differences can have big implications as far as the amount of weight you lose, how quickly you lose it, and how your body looks.

All calories are not created equal

If you are going to be reducing your calorie intake, it's really important to do it in such a way that you build up your muscle mass at the same time. What you should do is to simply decide to eat the right calories. You're going to be consuming calories anyway, why not consume calories that build up your muscle and reduce your body fat?

When you drastically decrease the amount of carbohydrate calories you eat and switch to mostly protein calories, you end up burning the weight loss candle from both ends. Not only do you reduce the amount of calories you eat daily, so you are more likely to achieve a net negative calorie state, you also eat food that produces a larger and leaner muscle mass. The net effect you get is awesome: you weigh less and look better. Pretty neat, right?

First, get an understanding of what you're working with

I mentioned earlier that your body is constantly burning calories even if you're not exercising.

When you're not exercising, your body still needs to burn calories to stay alive. On top of this, you're also burning calories in line with your regular lifestyle. The amount of calories you burn to remain alive is called your Basal Metabolic Rate (BMR). It measures the minimum calories you need to handle your body's most basic activities like cell production, digestion, blood circulation, and breathing. Since this is very specific to your body's most basic activities, the most accurate way to determine your BMR calorie requirements is through very precise and specific lab testing. Most people don't have access to such testing nor would most people shell out the necessary bucks to get such a highly accurate medical-grade reading.

Given the realities above, for practical purposes, the "BMR" readings people get (through their own calculations using a formula or with online calculators) is actually, their resting metabolic rate. This is the total amount of calories your body burns when it is at rest. This measurement is usually taken after a full night's rest first thing in the morning. Keep in mind that this reading is reflective of your lifestyle and existing muscle mass. It doesn't measure the bare minimum calories you need to stay alive. Still, it makes for a great stand-in for your BMR.

To get your BMR, you can use one of the many online BMR calculators available on the Net or you can use the formula below: The most common equation used is Harris-Benedict

For Men: BMR = 88.362 + (13.397 x weight in kg) + (4.799 x height in cm) - (5.677 x years of age)

For Women: BMR = 447.593 + (9.247 x weight in kg) + (3.098 x height in cm) - (4.330 x years of age)

Get your BMR since you'll use that as a base line for your meal plans.

Calculate your TDEE

TDEE stands for Total Daily Energy Expenditure. This number is based on your BMR but with one modification: you factor in your actual typical day's activity level. This figures your actual practical daily calorie requirements. When you eat less calories than your TDEE, you start to lose weight. How quickly and how much weight you lose depends on the net negative calorie state you reach.

To calculate TDEE use the following formula:

TDEE = BMR x Activity Factor

Select your activity level below and multiply that number by your BMR to get your TDEE

Activity Intensity Multiplier Table

Sedentary
Little to no Exercise/ desk job

TDEE = 1.2 x BMR

Light activity
Light exercise or sports 1 – 3 days/ week
TDEE = 1.375 x BMR

Moderate activity
Moderate Exercise or sports 3 – 5 days/ week
TDEE = 1.55 x BMR

Highly active
Heavy Exercise or sports 6 – 7 days/ week
TDEE = 1.725 x BMR

Extremely high activity
Very heavy exercise/ physical job/ training twice a day
TDEE = 1.9 x BMR

TDEE will yield the minimum calories you need to eat daily to maintain your weight. If you want to lose weight, eat less calories than the TDEE amount.

Counting your calories, the quick and easy way

Since calorie intake is crucial to weight loss, you need to be as meticulous and accurate as possible regarding the food you're eating. You can't simply "eyeball" the servings of the food you're eating. You might actually be eating too much calories that it can make weight loss difficult. You should use digital scales and measuring cups to ensure that you're eating the right quantity of food. Accuracy is crucial!

Accurate measurement is also crucial to determining the amount of protein you're putting in your diet daily. The key to getting ripped is to consume enough protein every day while minimizing carbohydrates and other compounds that increase blood sugar. You can't use guesstimates. You can't just rely on your taste buds because they have a way of fooling you. You end up eating too much that you don't achieve a net negative calorie state.

Chapter 3

How to control your hunger for more sustainable weight loss

There are several ways to control hunger. I am not going to insist on one particular method because everybody's different with different tastes and experiences. You may have different preferences. Plus, I'm not really in the position to tell you that you need to eat in a particular way because it is a one-size-fits-all solution to all weight loss issues. Instead, I'm just going to lay out several alternative approaches you can take. You can either choose to follow all of these, some or almost none of them. Whatever the case is, you need to follow the tips that would produce the best results in your situation.

First, try loading up one more protein. When you eat protein-dense foods, you feel fuller longer because there's usually enough fat packed in that package. Your brain feels fuller in and satiated for a longer period. The amount of calories you take in are also much lower than if you were to eat carbohydrate-rich foods.

Carbohydrates work with your blood sugar to determine your hunger levels. You end up eating more carb – rich foods than if you were to stick to a mostly protein diet. Just as important, when you switch to a protein-heavy diet, you can build your muscle mass or preserve the muscle mass that you already have.

Load up on fiber-rich foods

Eating foods that have a higher amount of dietary fiber helps you feel fuller for longer period. Fiber swells when mixed with the water in your stomach. This stretches your stomach. Your stomach then sends satiety signals to your brain and this leads to your brain releasing satiety hormones throughout your system. The bottom line is that you end up eating less and this, of course, reduces your total calorie intake.

Eating fiber-rich foods also helps clean up your system which leads to a more pronounced feeling of being full. This is especially true with high-fiber foods which contain more guar gum and pectin. Another great benefit of high-fiber foods is that they often carry a lot of vitamins, loaded with minerals and quite a bit of antioxidants. Not only do you eat fewer calories but you feel fuller and enjoy better health overall.

Another great way to lose weight with your simple food source strategies is to **eat more solids than liquids**. When you consume a primarily liquid diet, your brain tries to compensate by craving solid foods. This happens most frequently when you drink liquid snacks.

According to research studies, a diet consisting primarily of solid snacks led to lesser intense feelings of hunger and lower desire to consume food overall. You feel fuller for longer period. This is due to the fact that solid foods require more of your digestive processes that send out fullness signals. Also, when you chew on your food, your taste buds send signals that promote feelings of satiety.

Drinking coffee can also make you feel fuller for a longer period.

It stimulates the release of a peptide called YY. This hormone has been linked feelings of fullness and satiety. The more coffee you drink, the less hungry you feel. Interestingly enough, it's not the caffeine that triggers the reduction in hunger signals. According to research studies, decaf coffee works even better than regular coffee in producing this feeling of fullness for as much as three hours.

Drink more water

By drinking more water, you can decrease the level of hunger pangs/cravings you feel in between meals. Also, you need to drink quite a bit of water to aid your liver in turning fats into energy. It's a good idea to drink a zero-calorie beverage like water before a meal so that you can eat less calories during the meal. You end up boosting your satiety signals longer.

View Eating as an Experience

Most people just go through their meals like chores. Most people would rather keep on doing what they're doing at work or at home without having to stop and eat. Of course that's impossible, so most of us just zip through our meals. This really is too bad because if you are serious about losing weight, you need to stop, experience, pay more attention to and fully appreciate what you're doing.

Eating is not just one of those things that you need to do everyday. It's not like you are walking to the mailbox to pick up mail or any other type of routine activity. It can be a celebration of taste. It can be a truly rewarding experience that reminds you what it means to be truly alive. While it may be impractical to say to everybody that this should be your attitude towards eating, paying more attention to what you eat can pay off tremendously when it comes to losing weight. Try to eat in a mindful way, just look at your meal as an experience. Don't rush through it, allow yourself to fully experience the tastes and textures of your meal.

The net effect of this is that you would tend to eat less, but feel more satisfied. By simply deciding to eat more mindfully, you end up eating less. This goes a long way in reducing your overall calorie intake. Additionally, when you eat more mindfully, you decrease hunger, and you feel fuller longer. This also helps you avoid binge eating.

Eat More Dark Chocolates

According to research studies, dark chocolate contains some chemical compounds that actually suppress appetite. Interestingly enough, if you eat enough dark chocolate, your cravings for sweets actually decrease. In addition to this, researchers have found that the stearic acid dark chocolate contains, actually slows down the digestion process, the net effect is that you feel fuller for a longer period of time. There is also very interesting research which suggests that simply smelling dark chocolate can help you achieve the same effect. According to one particular study, noted that the simple act of smelling chocolate made up of 85% dark chocolate, suppressed hunger and appetite hormones.

Eat More Ginger

If you're into Chinese food and other Asian cuisine, you probably already have your fill of ginger. However, if you normally eat food that doesn't contain ginger, you might want to consider this ingredient. It not only packs quite a bit of health benefits like anti-inflammatory and blood sugar regulation qualities, it also helps your body modulate hunger signals. You feel less hungry if you eat a token amount of ginger everyday. According to one study, drinking a simple ginger tea made up of hot water and 2 grams of ginger for breakfast, reduces hunger after this meal.

Eat More Spicy Food

Certain foods help you feel fuller longer. When you eat foods that are high in Capsaicin, which are normally found in peppers, your hunger signals are recalibrated. You'll also feel fuller for a longer period of time.

There is also research that suggests that the extra heat generated by both hot and sweet peppers elevates the number of calories your body burns after a meal. Don't bet the bank on this though, the increased calorie burn is very slight, but if you're like most people struggling with their weight, every little bit helps.

Trick Your Eyes

Overeating is really a result of processing sensory signals. Your brain is always sending signals to your body. Your perception drives how hungry you feel. When you trick yourself by eating food on smaller plates, your mind is more open to thinking that it's eaten enough. You can actually feel quite full eating smaller and smaller portions using smaller plates. According to one study, people who were given large bowls to, gave themselves larger servings. Compare these with other study participants who gave themselves smaller servings because they had smaller plates and bowls to work with. These all works unconsciously and this can help you eat less and feel fuller for a much longer period of time.

The same applies to using a bigger fork. When you have a big fork, and you are able to pick up more food, you actually serve yourself less food. Why? You feel that you're already giving yourself enough food. According to a study comparing small forks and big forks, participants who were using small forks often felt that they had to compensate for the smaller size of their forks by eating more. The differential can be as large as close to 15 percent.

Workout More

By simply hitting the gym, you can retrain your body's hunger signals. Not only can you lose weight by increasing the rate at which your body burns calories, but exercise also releases hormones throughout your system, that increases the feeling of fullness and satiety.

According to research studies, both resistance exercises or weight training and aerobic exercises are effective in affecting hunger hormone levels. This leads to smaller meal sizes after exercising. If you're looking to feel less hungry, it's a good idea to start your day with moderate exercise and then exercise again near the evening.

Sleep More

Sleeping longer can actually reduce your hunger signals. First, your fullness or satiety hormones are recharged while you sleep. The more sleep you get, the slightly you would be hungry throughout the day. Second, when you sleep, your will power is increased. You can end up making better eating decisions during your waking hours.

Manage Your Cortisol by Managing Stress

Cortisol is the stress hormone your body releases when it feels pressure. If you're under a lot of stress, there is a lot of cortisol in your bloodstream. This elevated level leads to greater hunger signals. Studies have shown that increased food cravings and hunger are linked with high cortisol levels. This factor doesn't work alone because when you're stressed out, your cortisol increases while at the same time, your peptide YY, which is a fullness hormone, is artificially decreased.

According to research studies, participants who were given a stressful test, tended to eat on average 22 percent more food than participants who were not given stress-inducing test. Reduce your stress levels to manage your food cravings and at the same time increase your sense of satiety. The overall effect is that you eat less, and your daily calorie intake goes down.

Snack on more Proteins

Protein-dense foods tend to be quite effective in managing hunger. If you use protein-heavy foods like yogurt or peanuts for snacks, you moderate your hunger throughout the day. The best part is since these are calorie-dense, you won't need too much of them to feel full. A little goes a long way. Eating snacks that are packed with protein, suppresses your hunger and might actually help you cut down on the size of your next meal.

Chapter 4

Shopping Your Way to a Slimmer Waistline

Now that you have a guide and some practical tips on how to manage your hunger signals throughout the day, the next step is to line up your shopping habits with your weight loss goals. Did you know that the way you shop can impact your weight? People who tend to overeat, tend to shop a certain way. By simply paying more attention to your shopping habits, you can take care of a very important detail that might be undermining your weight loss efforts all this time.

The Worst Shopping Habit

The worst thing that you could is to go to the grocery store with no list. You're basically at the mercy of your senses when you do that. You have to understand that modern grocery stores and retail chains use a lot of psychology to maximize customers' per store visit. This strategy does not have your best interest in mind as far as your weight goes.

It's a good idea to make sure that you plan out your shopping trips properly so you can reduce your calorie intake. Keep the following tips in mind to help you shop your way to a lower weight.

Plan out Low-Calorie High-Protein Meals

Before you even think of going to the store make sure you have a clear idea of what kind of meals you would like to eat during the week. This includes, of course, snacks. Just list out the names of these dishes.

Next, create a rough meal plan out of them and list out their ingredients. Plan meals efficiently by focusing on common ingredients or core ingredients. Not only does this help you to buy in bulk which can help you save quite a few dollars, it also highlights the importance of certain ingredients. If you notice that there are too many carbohydrate-rich or sugar-based ingredients in your list, you might need to change your meal plan. By drilling down and breaking up dishes based on their common ingredients, you can make better meal selection decisions.

Cook in Bulk

It's also a good idea to prepare low-calorie high-protein meals in bulk. Let's face it; most of us don't have the luxury of time. Most of us would rather zip in and out of our apartments or houses. Most Americans after all, have a busy lifestyle.

It's a good idea to cook in bulk because you save a lot of energy and time doing so. You also are forced to plan ahead. You don't burn up as much will power trying to decide which meal to prepare for which day. Everything is already laid out. As long as you have the right storage containers for your fridge, you're set for several days. This saves a lot of time and most importantly; it saves a lot of will power on your part.

The less effort you spend making choices, the more will power you can devote to resisting temptation or making often inconvenient decisions like hitting the gym consistently.

Your Grocery Shopping Habits Impact your Weight Loss Chances

Make no mistake about it, the way you shop at the grocery has a direct impact on your waistline. You need to make sure that you plan out everything ahead of time. You need to make sure that all details are taken care of. As I mentioned previously, you need to avoid putting yourself in a situation where you're just blindly pulling stuff of the shelf. This is a one-way street to unwanted pounds. There are going to be all sorts of brightly-colored packages and well-designed boxes and cans all intended to appeal to your senses. They're all intended for you to load up and buy stuff you wouldn't otherwise buy.

Prepare for Batch Food Cooking

One very important tip I picked up along the way is to set up a regular schedule for preparing food, cooking, and going to the grocery store. Even if you're the busiest person you know, as long as you have a regular schedule for doing these three things, you can prepare food in the most time-effective way possible.

You don't have to put yourself in the uncomfortable position of opening your fridge door and seeing that your foods' ingredients are not prepared for cooking. A lot of people stumble with their weight loss plan when they put themselves in this position. What do you think they would do? That's right-they would head straight to a fast food joint, and overeat. This happens all the time!

Instead of painting yourself in a corner this way, set up a schedule where you go to a grocery store, pick up ingredients, prepare those ingredients and then cook them at certain times of the week. In this situation, when you open the fridge door, and you see that all the ingredients for your meals are already chopped up and prepared, you can then just take several plastic containers, open them, put them in a pot, and quickly prepare your meal. Whether you're doing stir fries, preparing steak, and all points in between, this method of preparing food in advance, can help you stay on track as far as your weight loss plans go. Again, I can't emphasize this enough. Don't put yourself in a situation where you feel that it takes too much effort to prepare food. The more you can clean up, chop up, and slice and dice food ahead of time, the better off you would be. You will end up giving yourself excuses, for going to a fast food restaurant.

I need to mention one key tip here though, make sure that when you are preparing ahead of time, make cooking as easy as possible. What I mean is your ingredients must be prepared in such a way that you basically just have to mix them or heat them. You then have yourself a quick and yummy meal. Don't just stick to preliminary preparation like, for example, peeling carrots. Dice and slice them for easier cooking. Don't just stick with the basics.

Special Tip for Preparing Meat

Meat can be a hassle to prepare especially if you're just storing slabs of it in your freezer. Make things easier on yourself by chopping meat into meal-size portions. Second, cook these until they are 70-80 percent done. Next, store them in your fridge-don't store them in your freezer.

When you're ready to cook them, you only need to take them out of their plastic containers, mix them with your veggies and other ingredients, and you have yourself a quick meal. Don't put yourself in a tight spot where you have to thaw meat from the freezer before you can chop it up. Even if you chopped up meat, and you froze it, this is still too much of a hassle.
Again, you want to set things up so that they are hassle-free as possible. The less cooking time, the better. So, precooked meat and certain types of fish, definitely go a long way in helping you cut down the cooking time while maximizing convenience.

Chapter 5

Make Sure You Use the Right Equipment when Bulking Up

Since you're looking to both lose weight and bulk up your muscles, you need to make sure you have the right equipment. The big danger most people in your position come across, is they try to eyeball things. They look at a portion of food ingredients and go with their gut feeling, whether it's the right amount to eat. That's a one-way street to weight gain. You may lose some weight here and there but ultimately, you're fighting a losing battle. Since you're not meticulous about the specific amount of calories, you're eating in any given day, the danger of overeating will be just too high.

Avoid overeating by being precise about your serving sizes and ingredient portions as possible. Here are some pieces of equipment that you need to pick up to maximize your success.

Digital scales

Digital scales are awesome because they're easy to figure out. There's no guesswork needed. When you put ingredients into a tray, and you place it on your digital scale, you get the proper weight-instantly. You don't have to make judgment calls regarding the lines of an analog scale. Also, digital scales are more sensitive, so you have a higher assurance that the weight that it reports is actually accurate. This is crucial because pinpoint accuracy is needed for maximum calorie control and planning. You're trying to cut down on your calorie intake so you can achieve a negative state for weight loss. There is a very little room for error. Digital scales make it easy for you to figure out just exactly how much calories you are ingesting every single day.

Measuring Cups

Measuring cups are important because they also help you avoid "eyeballing" recipes. When you play fast and loose regarding ingredient amounts, you might actually be loading up on extra unwanted calories to your meals. I know this may seem a bit too meticulous for some people but the good news is, as long as you keep using measuring cups, it quickly becomes a habit.

In fact, from my experience, I kept using measuring cups regularly that I reached a point where I feel that I was going to screw up the recipe if I did not use the proper measuring cups. The bottom line is tight measurements enable to scale down your portions to where they need to be. If you're going to be reducing your serving sizes for calorie reduction, you definitely need all the help you can get. Measuring cups enable you to accurately scale down your calorie intake by reducing your ingredients' portions.

Store Food like a Champ

Convenience is crucial to your diet. I hope that much is clear. Again, as I mentioned in the previous chapter, you don't want to put yourself in a situation where you open your fridge door and you are intimidated by the amount of work you need to do to turn those raw ingredients into a meal. By the same token, you don't want to be demotivated by the fact that you have to wait for all this meat to thaw just so you can cook yourself a meal.

The secret, as I mentioned in Chapter 4, is to prepare all these different ingredients ahead of time. In the case of meat and fish, it's a good idea to cook them partially before you fully cook them. You cook them partially and store them. This way, when you're ready to cook your meal, you just need to take out the right ingredient containers, mix them together, and you're done. You save a tremendous amount of time. This also helps leaves you psychologically motivated.

Eating lower calorie meals is not only feasible and advised, but convenient. To make this happen, you need to have the right equipment to store food like a champ. Load up on Tupperware or similar brands. These food containers are great because they're stackable, and they're very ergonomic as far as your fridge space goes. It's important that you pick food containers that have a tight lock mechanism. Since you're going to be storing food for as much as maybe two weeks, you need to make sure that moisture and air are kept out. There are many different Tupperware designs that create a vacuum seal. The moment you put food in there, and you close the lid; the air is locked so you don't have to worry about the moisture seeping in.

The proper equipment also helps to ensure that you save money. Why? By ensuring your food doesn't spoil, pretty straightforward. Keep in mind that you need to buy quite a bit of this equipment because you're going to be breaking up your meal plan into small modular ingredient portions. This is crucial to your ten-minute meal plan. You have to prepare all food items together as much as possible and store them in small modular containers. This way, you don't run the risk of spoiling a batch of ingredients when you're just cooking up a single meal. By having many different Tupperware or plastic containers containing enough ingredients for one meal, and stacking them and storing them efficiently, you can prepare meals more efficiently and conveniently.

Unleash the Power of a George Foreman Grill

When it comes to preparing meat and certain types of vegetables, the George Foreman grill is a godsend. It truly is. It has a classic design that allows for quick electric grilling. It emits less smoke, it can be used indoors in many cases, it drains fat easily, and it allows for targeted cooking. The best part is cleaning up after a meal. It doesn't have to be a hassle.

You just let the grill cool down, and you use a damp cloth to wipe the surface of the grill, and you're done. Disassembling the grill for more thorough cleaning is also quick and convenient. I can't recommend the George Foreman grill enough. If you're serious about cooking your meals in a quick, easy, and highly convenient way, this should be part of your cooking arsenal. It's almost non-negotiable.

How to Pick the Right Pressure Cooker

One definitely non-negotiable piece of equipment for the single guy looking to bulk up and lose weight is a pressure cooker. A pressure cooker is non-negotiable because it is able to cook meat in a ridiculously short period of time. You have to understand, typically for stews, we're talking as much as upwards of three hours to cook down blocks of meat. With the right pressure cooker and properly prepared small cubes of precooked meat, you can reduce the cooking time to mere minutes. This enables you to cook more yummy food in no time.

When picking among pressure cooker designs, you need to focus on size. Also, you need to pay attention to the design of the pressure cooker. Some use a whistle type system to tell you that your meal is ready. Others have other methods of letting you know. It's a good idea to pay attention to these differences and pick the features that fit your lifestyle the best. The key consideration of course is convenience. The pressure cooker should make cooking meat as convenient and easy as possible.

Chapter 6

Quick Cooking Methods for Dudes

For the single guy, cooking can be a thankless and annoying chore. I really can't blame them because most guys used to run away from their moms when mom wanted their help around the kitchen. For many guys, this is kind of a built-in reaction. I don't blame them at all. The good news is there are cooking methods that are quick, easy, require zero-to-low skill, and relatively painless. By simply investing some time into these cooking methods, you can prepare yummy satisfying meals in no time. Cooking doesn't have to be a chore. Cooking doesn't have to be a hassle.

Salads

The big advantage of preparing salads, is that they are quick and versatile. Also, when you're preparing salads, you also are given a tremendous opportunity to load up on ingredients that are very good for you. I'm talking about green leafy vegetables and chopped veggies.
To prepare a salad, you just need to chop up the ingredients, put them together, add some dressing and then, toss everything together. This is very quick, very easy, and depending on your ingredients and dressing, very tasty.

The big drawback, is that you can easily fall into a rut. You can end up doing the same thing over and over again as far as ingredient and dressing selections go. Some guys try to cheat by using very fatty dressings. Worse, some guys use dressings that are heavy in sugar. Since you're trying to gain muscle while losing weight, your focus should be increasing your protein and lean fat intake. The best way to do this is to be very careful regarding your salad choices. Load up more on protein-heavy veggies like broccoli.

Skillet Dishes

A lot of guys love skillet dishes because you take one skillet, put all your ingredients in there, apply heat, and you're done. It's self-contained, quick, and easy. Plus, it's very easy to clean up after yourself because you just have a skillet and a plate. It doesn't take long for you to just scrub down and clean up these items after a meal.

The big disadvantage to skillet dishes is that you need to pick recipes that can be cooked in one self-contained unit. You have to pick dishes that don't require different stages of cooking. Some cuisines are friendlier to skillet cooking. Others are notorious for multi-stage cooking. You take a raw ingredient; you cook it, and then the process it. Then, you take another raw ingredient, cook it, and process it. Then, you process them together, and then you wait for some time and then; you serve. Nobody has the time to do all that. Skillet dishes enable you to do everything all at once with one cooking equipment. Unfortunately, not all cuisines are as friendly to skillet cooking as others.

Skewer Meals and Stoked Up Grilling

If you're a meat eater, skewer meals are awesome. If you like kebabs, this is the way to go. Even if you're a vegetarian, you can use this cooking method to cook great-tasting grilled veggies. Skewer meals are tremendous. Not only can skewering and stove-top grilling save you time, they also preserve and seal in the flavor of the ingredients you're cooking. Best of all, it's easy to clean up because you just swipe debris off the grill, wipe down with a damp rag, and you're good to go.

The best disadvantage to skewer meals is oftentimes you have to marinate. While this is not a problem for most dishes, it can be a problem if you are going to be preparing many different marinated dishes at once. This is a headache because you might end up mixing flavors. I'm of course talking about different types of meat using different types of marinades. Another issue that you need to keep in mind is the smoking factor. Grilling gives off smoke and, depending on your living accommodations, this can put a tremendous amount of pressure on your ventilation system if your grill fan is not in tip-top shape. You might end up with very smoky or smelly rooms in your home. The best solution for grilling smoke? Grill outdoors if you can.

Stir Frying

In ancient China, according to legend, cooking fuel was scarce, so the ancient Chinese had to come up with a cooking method that concentrated all the heat in a small area of a pan to cut down on cooking time. Thus, the wok was born.

Stir frying is all about wok cooking.

You pre-chop all the ingredients and prepare your sauce. Add oil to the wok and put the different ingredients one by one. Add the sauce, heat it up, keep stirring, and you're done in a very short of time. Whether you like fried rice, or Mongolian beef, or Kung Pao chicken and all points in between, stir frying saves a lot of time. Most importantly, it produces very tasty food.

It's also very easy to clean up after stir-frying because you only need to take your wok, and fill it with water, wait for it to boil and then quickly scrape, and you're done. It doesn't take much time to do stir frying. The best of all, stir frying is actually one of the most versatile forms of cooking because you could pretty much throw any combination of ingredients as long as you know the flavor profile you are aiming for. You can come up with great-tasting dishes quickly.

The big disadvantage to stir frying is that like salads, it's easy to get caught in a rut. It's easy to basically prepare the same stir fry dish day after day. Make sure to break this boredom. Make sure to mix up your sauces. Try to experiment. There are all sorts of textures that you could play with. There are also all sorts of scents you can go for. A dash of sesame seed oil can add a very welcome exotic element to your otherwise straightforward stir fried meals.

Steaks

When it comes to ease, steaks win hands down every single time. It's probably the easiest way to cook meat in a serious way. You just need to slice the meat to the right thickness, slap it on a grill or pan and you're in business! It's almost foolproof.

With all that said, there is such a thing as passable steak (which most guys settle for) and the best steak. This is the bad news. If you're looking to cook the very best steaks at home, you need to invest quite a bit of time. It takes quite a few tries to get it perfect. You also need to experiment with different sauces and rubs or marinades for optimal taste. The good news is that, if you're just looking for great-tasting food quickly, cooking steaks is the way to go. Now, if you're looking for the perfect steaks or really high-quality steaks, then you need to invest time.

The Secret to Juicy, Time-saving, and Effective Cooking for Single Guys

If you're a single dude looking to maximize your time and also ensure yourself of the best food, here's the secret. The secret is quite simple: Mix things up. I've already laid out some very powerful cooking methods in this chapter. You need to just jump from one method to the next. By mixing up salads, skillets, skewers, stir fries, and steaks, you add a tremendous amount of variety to your meal plan, and this ensures you never get bored. What you're trying to avoid is to put yourself in a situation where you feel so intimidated by cooking, or you feel so bored by the food that you have, that you end up taking a trip to a fast food joint.

Chapter 7

Plan your Meals for Maximum Time Management

Different foods require different cooking time. Be aware of this central fact. You have to square your schedule with this reality. Otherwise, it's too easy to again, find yourself in the tight spot where you feel compelled to go to McDonald's or Taco Bell because you don't have the time to cook. Be aware of variations in your schedule. As I mentioned in Chapter 4, it's a good idea to prepare things in advance.

Precook your meats and store them for easy and quick preparation. Again, our time budget here is ten minutes per meal. Accordingly, it's a good idea to cook ahead of time and store them. The big danger is that you need up with bad cooking because you haven't budgeted enough time. The biggest danger, of course, is for you to just give up on everything and just head to a fast food joint for maximum convenience. Do that enough times, and you can kiss your diet goodbye.

How do you plan your meals for maximum time management?

Cook Grains Ahead of Time

You have to remember time that cooking grains takes a relatively long period of time. Whether we're talking about quinoa or rice, or any other grain, for that matter, they take a quite bit of time. They require boiling, and many grains require steaming. To fix this problem, cook gains in batches. If you eat a lot of rice, get a large rice cooker, cook up all that rice and then split up the steamed rice into smaller Tupperware containers. These batches ensure you one complete rice meal or package. Best of all, you only need to heat them in the microwave or stir fry the rice for a very short of time on your stove.

Considerations in Cooking Meat

Cooking meat is faster, but it can also be very tricky. You see; certain types of meat are very easy to burn. Seafood, for example, is notoriously easy to overcook. I've had the sad experience of overcooking squid rings. With squid, and for that matter, octopus, if you go past a certain amount of cooking time, the texture of squid and octopus feels exactly like rubber. Consider yourself warned. Accordingly, you have to under cook these foods for later full cooking. You need to be mindful of the precise cooking times of the meat and seafood ingredients you're working with. Again, cooking seafood is the trickiest. Cooking the best steak is cake-walk compared to getting seafood just right.

Cooking Veggies

There are many ways to cook vegetables. Veggie preparation runs the gamut from boiling to stewing to grilling and baking. Stewed vegetables are the most error-tolerant. If you spend too much time or spend too little time, you can still get away with great taste.

Other veggies are not as tolerant. For example, if you're looking for a crisp texture, you need to pay more attention to tiny details, otherwise, you're going to get soggy veggies or veggies that are raw.

The Most Important Tip for Cooking Stews

If you're cooking stewed dishes, here's the best advice I could give you. You have two factors you're working with. You're dealing with either heat level or cooking length. These work in inverse proportions. For example, if you're stuck with low heat, then you need to increase cooking time. Conversely, if you don't have that much time for cooking, you can increase the heat to speed up cooking. It also helps if you soaked beans overnight.

Stews are great because they're usually harder to screw up. To screw up stews, you have to make the wrong judgment calls as far as ingredients are concerned. When it comes to the actual cooking process, stewing is more error-tolerant than other methods of cooking.

Chapter 8

Mixing and Matching your Meal Plan's Items

Variety as, they say, is the spice of life. If you're a single guy looking to hit the gym and get buff while losing weight through dieting, listen up. As I mentioned previously, it's very to get stuck in a rut. It's very easy to look at your diet as consisting of a tight range of dishes that form you "go to" foods. Well, don't fall for this trap. The more bored you get, the higher the likelihood you will get off your diet and start packing on the pounds. That's just the harsh reality you have to deal with.

You need to keep your body engaged by putting as much variety into your meal plans. This is easy to get but the problem is, implementation. You see; different foods have different nutrient profiles. If you're not careful, you might be loading up on foods that short circuit your weight loss efforts and plans. Understand how important characteristics of these food categories so you can make the proper planning decisions.

Proteins

Proteins can come from meat and non-meat sources. There are high-protein vegetables like broccoli. As much as possible your diet should focus almost primarily on proteins. Not only do protein-rich foods help you build up your muscle mass so you can look more toned and fit, they also pack calories that make you feel fuller longer. This has the very helpful effect of cutting down on your hunger cravings throughout the day.

All this takes some getting used to. It's not like you just load up on proteins and then all of a sudden, your daily calorie intake crashes onto the floor. It doesn't work that way. It's something that you ease into gradually. The good news is that there is such a variety of protein sources out there that you can plan to cook up diverse yummy meals that gradual calorie reduction becomes a tasty experience.

Carbohydrates

Carbohydrates are found in foods that have starch or sugar. The unpleasant reality of carbohydrates is that all vegetables have varying levels of carbohydrates. Some have more; others have way less. But they all have carbohydrates. What I'm trying to say is that you really cannot cut out carbohydrates completely from your diet. You can only manage it to a low enough level that it doesn't short circuit your weight loss plans.

Why is carbohydrate control crucial? As I mentioned previously, you want to train your body to burn your fat as an energy source instead of doing what it normally does. In normal situations, your body will burn up sugar and carbohydrates as its primary source of energy.
This has tremendously negative implications as far as hunger management goes because if your body goes through pronounced blood sugar fluctuations, you're basically stuck in a position where you're hungry pretty much throughout the day. You don't want that to happen. Pick foods that have low carbohydrate levels and high-protein content.

Fats

Fats can be found in your diet in two forms either oils (concentrated or locked in nuts/seeds) or fat found with animal protein. Fats are not as demonic as we have previously been led to believe. In fact, the National Institutes of Health in the United States, has recently overhauled its dietary recommendations regarding fats. It's no longer the bogeyman of meal planning. Why? Loading up on fat actually can help the ketosis process along.

When you eat foods that are high in fat, you start training your body to burn fat for fuel instead of the sugar in your bloodstream. This is important for the guys looking to lose weight while building up muscle mass. The plan is to train your body to burn stored fat first so the fat layers are peeled away, and the underlying muscle mass is shown. This will make you look more toned and fit. Also, you feel less hungry.

The "ignition switch" to this ketogenic process is a healthy amount of fat in the form of avocados or coconut oil, spices.

Spices can be very helpful but in small amounts. You really can't have a spice-only diet. That's going to be very hard on your palate. With that said, spices can bring a lot of flavor to your meals, and if you end, in the case of peppers, can actually spur the fat-burning process. This is called the 'thermogenic' reaction where your body's cells' temperature is increased so you burn more calories. Not only do spices help trigger this process, but they also infuse a lot of flavor into your meals.

Vegetables

It's important to always include vegetables in your meal plans. Not only do vegetables contain a great amount of nutrients and vitamins; they also contain antioxidants. Antioxidants appear to help the body fight off cancer and other diseases. Veggies also bring a lot of flavor variety into the table. So, if you're looking to mix things up, load up on the veggies. The good news is, veggies aren't just all carbohydrates. In fact, there are vegetables that have high fiber, high protein and low carbohydrates. Load up on high-protein vegetables like broccoli so you can get that lean, toned muscular body sooner rather than later.

Chapter 9

HIIT weight training

If you're looking to lose a lot of weight while toning down drastically, you need to shift your exercise strategy to HIIT. It stands for high-intensity interval training. Make no mistake about it; using this exercise strategy can build up your muscle mass for higher resting calorie burn. Why is this a big deal?

Well, as I mentioned previously in this book, simply walking around and doing your everyday exercises require energy. Your body is always burning up calories. This is called your resting calorie burn. However, if you want to take it to a much higher level, you need to build up your muscle mass. The larger your muscles get, the more energy they require.

Also, when you work out at the gym, do weightlifting and resistance exercises, microscopic tears occur all over your muscle mass. This, of course leads, to sore muscles. This also increases the amount of calories your body needs daily for tissue repair. Put these two factors together and you can take your resting calorie burn rate to a much higher level.

The great news

The great news about building up your muscle mass for a higher passive burn rate, is that it doesn't have to take too much effort. It definitely does not take much time. A lot of people think that to get buff, you need to pump iron at the gym for hours on end. This is absolutely not true; thanks to HIIT, you can spend as little as 20 minutes at the gym and have a lot to show for it. In fact, you don't even need to go to the gym if you just want to do HIIT. Not only can you get buffed as quickly as possible but you can also save up on gym membership fees.

What does HIIT involve

As previously mentioned, HIIT is high-intensity interval training. You take some weight lifting, resistance exercise or cardio exercise in budget short periods of time. This can be as little as 20 minutes every day. You then break up these 20 minutes into smaller blocks. For example, 20 minutes can be broken up into five blocks of four minutes. These blocks are set up where you exercise intensely for one block then follow it up with a resting period. After the resting period is over, you then exercise intensely and then rest.

It is important to keep in mind that HIIT is not about repetitions. When you normally do weightlifting, you focus on how many reps you do. In cardio exercises like treadmill, running or climbing exercises, you measure your progress based on distance. However, you can throw these measurements out of the window with HIIT. Instead, your only metric is how intense your workout is.

Most people measured this by how close they are to passing out or running out of breath. You obviously want to reach a high enough level of activity until you start running out of breath. You then dial things down a notch and keep it at that level. HIIT also accommodates scaling up your effort. The first time you try HIIT, you probably are not going to go all that far when you sprint. Maybe you probably wouldn't achieve too many reps if you're pumping weights. Still, by breaking up your workout time into these alternating blocks of high intensity exercises and resting periods, you can scale up your effort over time. You don't have to accomplish a lot overnight but as long as the intensity is there, the results will show in your mid-section or other flabby parts.

Many people on a low-carb high-protein diet reported drastic results when they paired their high protein-low carb diet with an HIIT exercise regimen.

Mix up your HIIT schedule

The secret to HIIT is to give yourself enough variety to scale up your intensity over time. One of the best ways to do this is to mix up the different types of training you can do. On the first day, you can do cardio exercises, then you can follow up with weight training, after that you can then do resistance training. You should also rest on the weekend.

If you mix things up using different types of exercises, you can achieve better results in a shorter period. It's also going to be much harder for you to burn out from your workout schedule because there's enough variety in your routine. It's easier to burn out when you are just doing cardio day after day. The same goes with weight training or weight resistance training.

Chapter 10

Timing your meals properly

If you're looking to actually maximize your weight loss using the information contained in this book, I can't recommend about timing your meals enough. You see, your body has a built-in schedule for burning calories. If you ignore this built-in body clock, your body's calorie burning schedule might be working against you. By simply timing your meals properly, you can let your body's internal calorie burning clock work alongside your dieting and exercise efforts.

There are two ways to do it. You can use intermittent fasting or you can schedule your meals earlier in the day. There is no one perfect answer. Different people have different metabolisms and different preferences. You might want to try both of these techniques out and see which works better in your situation.

Unleashing the power of intermittent fasting

Did you know that you are already fasting? I know that in the minds of most people, when somebody mentions the word "fasting," they think of some sort of monk on top of a hill who doesn't eat for months. The truth is, whenever you go to sleep, you are already fasting technically speaking.

Intermittent fasting is fast gaining popularity because people discovered that by simply extending the daily period where they don't eat any calories at all, they can enjoy significant weight loss. The starting based of your fasting period, of course, is the time when you are asleep.

When you're sleeping, by definition, you're not eating. You take this period and stretch it. There are different "flavors" of intermittent fasting. Some require you to not eat for a whole day; others require you to eat only within a small time window. I'm not going to go into the details of these different ways do intermittent fasting. I just want to open your mind to the fact that this is one possible way for you to turbocharge the results that you're getting out from the rest of the tips shared in this book.

If you do it correctly, it's going to trigger a net negative calorie intake. The longer the time block, the more you segregate calorie intake. This can lead to greater weight loss. One particularly important way is to specifically skip a meal. There's a bit of a lively debate as to which meal to cut. Some people are sold on the idea that breakfast should be taken off the table. Others are convinced that dinner is purely optional and should be cut out.

Again, it all boils down to preferences. It also boils down to your comfort level. Regardless of how you play it, intermittent fasting works because you can time your calorie intake in such a way that it coincides with the time of day you are burning up calories the most. In my experience, cutting dinner the needs to better results because you wouldn't want to be eating calories precisely at the point in the day where your system starts to slow down and your body's beginning to unwind where you don't burn calories as efficiently as earlier in the day.

Of course, this all depends on your comfort level. Some people want to eat dinner. So if that's it is that your situation, then stick with dinner but you still need to dial down one of the other two meals in a typical day.

Schedule your meals early in the day

I've already alluded to this earlier. You would want to set up your meals in such a way that eating the bulk of your calories at precisely at the time of day where your body is burning up the most calories. Usually for most people with healthy metabolisms, this is in the morning or in the afternoon. It makes sense then to eat a big breakfast or a big lunch. It also makes sense to eat less for dinner or skip it entirely.

In the early evening and at night, your body's calorie burn rate winds down. You don't want to eat a lot of calories at night because a lot of these will get stored as fat. If you eat most of your calories in the form of a big breakfast or lunch, a lot of it will be burned up by your system earlier in the day. You get to eat more but feel less hungry throughout the day.

What is the secret? Cut down on sugar. Your body uses blood sugar as hunger signals. By cutting down on it, you will stabilize these signals and feel less hungry throughout the day.

The Recipes

1). Greek Yogurt w/ frozen blueberries and chocolate almonds

Ingredients:
1 cup Greek yogurt
1 cup frozen blueberries
11 chocolate covered almonds

Nutrition Facts:
Protein: 23g
Carbs: 40g
Fat: 13g
Total Calories: 369

How to Make It:
Put 1 cup of Greek yogurt in a bowl and add the frozen blueberries and chocolate covered almonds.

2). Steak with Vegetables and Sweet Potato

Ingredients:
1/2 pound of steak
1 medium sweet potato
2 cups of cruciferous vegetables (broccoli, brussel sprouts, kale, asparagus, etc.)

Nutrition Facts:
Protein: 64g
Carbs: 26g
Fat: 34g
Total Calories: 685

How to Make It:
Preheat oven to 450 degrees. Rub the steak with salt, pepper, and any other spices you want (I like Cajun). Place cast iron skillet on stove with high heat until pan is VERY hot. Let steak cook on each side for 90 seconds to cook each side. Place skillet into preheated oven for 2 minutes. When steak is done cooking, remove from oven and put it on a plate and cover with foil for 5 minutes – this will allow the steak to cook further and stay juicy.

Place the vegetables in the cast iron skillet with 1 tablespoon of oil (olive, coconut, etc.) and saute. Feel free to add spices.

Microwave sweet potato for 6-8 minutes (buy the microwavable kinds… duh!)

3). Buffalo Chicken Salad

Ingredients:
Lettuce, chopped
½ cup shredded carrots
4 tbsp ranch dressing
½ cup blue cheese crumbles
½ cup chicken breast
1 tablespoon vegetable oil, 1 turn of the pan
2 tablespoons butter
Salt and black pepper
1/4 cup hot sauce

Nutrition Facts:
Protein: 66g
Carbs: 5g
Fat: 46g
Total Calories: 700

How to Make It:
First preheat a skillet over medium heat. Add lettuce and carrots in a salad bowl. Put ranch dressing and blue cheese pieces in small bowl. Put the oil and butter in a hot pan and add the chicken pieces. Add salt and pepper and let the chicken sear for about 3 minutes then add hot sauce. Reduce the heat and cook 5 more minutes. Add dressing to salad and season with salt and pepper. Top the salad with Buffalo chicken and serve.

tried 1/3/2019

4). Taco Salad with Beans and Crushed Chips

Ingredients:

2 ripe tomatoes, diced
¼ cup sharp Cheddar, diced
1 large onion, diced
1 head iceberg lettuce, washed, drained and shredded
½ pound lean ground beef, browned, crumbled and drained
4 tbsp salad dressing (recommended: Catalina)
1 cup salsa

– beans

Nutrition Facts:

Protein: 47g
Carbs: 21g
Fat: 37g
Total Calories:

How to Make It:

Put ground beef in a hot skillet and sautee until it's brown. OR boil the ground beef and drain it (this gets rid of more fat from the meat)

Mix the tomatoes, cheese, onion, lettuce, and ground beef in a large bowl. Add the salad dressing and mix. Crush and add the chips just before serving and toss once more. Top each serving with salsa. Serve with tortilla chips or by itself.

5). Chicken and Veggie Stir Fry w/ Rice

Ingredients:
8 ounces chopped chicken breast
2 cups chopped broccoli
2 cups chopped cauliflower
½ chopped onion
½ carrot (optional, I'm not a big fan of carrots)
1 cup rice

Nutrition Facts:
Protein: 54g
Carbs: 45g
Fat: 8g
Total Calories: 485

How to Make It:
Stir fry all of the ingredients (chicken and vegetables) together with 1 tbsp of extra virgin olive oil or coconut oil and add salt, peppers and dried chili peppers as desired. Serve over rice. Add whatever kind of sauce you'd like.

6). Turkey Spinach Omelette

Ingredients:
½ cup onions
½ cup mushrooms
3 ounces turkey
6 egg whites
1 egg
1 slice low fat cheddar
1 cup spinach
2 pieces of toast (optional)

Nutrition Facts:
Protein: 54g
Carbs: 30g
Fat: 11g
Total Calories: 450

How to Make It:
Put the egg and egg whites in a bowl and add the other ingredients and mix them all up. Put them onto a frying pan with a small amount of oil and let it cook. Once it's done add the turkey slices and a slice of cheese and fold into an omelette.

7). Simple Spinach Scramble

Ingredients:
¼ cup onion (chopped)
½ cup mushrooms (chopped)
¼ cup green peppers (chopped)
1 cup spinach
6 egg whites
1 egg
2 pieces of toast (optional)

Nutrition Facts:
Protein: 33g
Carbs: 26g
Fat: 7g
Total Calories: 312

How to Make It:
Put the egg and egg whites in a bowl and add the other ingredients and mix them all up. Put them onto a frying pan with a small amount of oil and let it cook. Once it's done add I like to add spices on top or eat it with chili garlic sauce.

8). High Fiber Salmon Wraps

Ingredients:
1 can of canned salmon
1 tbsp olive oil mayo
Lemon juice (to taste)
Cumin (to taste)
Chili lemon pepper (to taste)
1 tbsp capers
Cilantro
High fiber wrap

Nutrition Facts:
Protein: 50g
Carbs: 20g
Fat: 22g
Total Calories: 450

How to Make It:
Add the canned salmon, mayo, spices, cilantro, and capers into a bowl and mix. Then add fresh lemon juice and spread it on a fiber wrap.

9). Whey Protein Mug Cake

Ingredients:
2 scoops whey protein powder
¼ cup instant pancake mix
1 tbsp chia seeds
Water (enough to make it soupy)
Whipped cream (optional)

Nutrition Facts:
Protein: 56g
Carbs: 43g
Fat: 11g
Total Calories: 490

How to Make It:
Put the protein powder, instant pancake mix, and chia seeds in a coffee mug and add enough water to make it a bit "liquidy". Then put it in the microwave for 2 minutes. Then let it cool for a minute and add some whipped cream to it.

It should look spongy and moist, if not, you need to add more water.

10). Breakfast Tacos

Ingredients:
1 tbsp salsa
2 corn tortillas
2 tbsp shredded cheddar cheese
½ cup liquid egg substitute

Nutrition Facts:
Protein: 19g
Carbs: 25g
Fat:6g
Total Calories: 225

How to Make It:
Put the salsa on the tortillas and add some cheese and put it all in the microwave until it melts. Warm a skillet over medium heat and add the egg substitute and mix until the eggs are cooked. Add it to the tortillas when you're done and eat them.

11). Orange Avocado Chicken Salad

Ingredients:
1 skinless, boneless chicken breast
2 cups mixed salad greens
¼ cup orange segments
¼ diced avocado
3 tbsp chopped red onion
1/8 tbsp cilantro-lime vinaigrette

Nutrition Facts:
Protein: 28g
Carbs: 10g
Fat: 24g
Total Calories: 367

How to Make It:
Chop the chicken breast into small pieces and broil it. Put the greens, avocado, onions, and chicken in a salad bowl and toss it with the vinaigrette.

12). Blackened Salmon Sandwich

Ingredients:
3 tbsp Cajun spice
Salt and pepper to taste
4 ounces salmon fillet
1 tbsp mayonnaise
1 tbsp olive oil
6-inch whole wheat ciabatta
2 slices of tomato
¼ cup shredded cabbage

Nutrition Facts:
Protein: 26g
Carbs: 30g
Fat: 32g
Total Calories: 518

How to Make It:
Warm up a non-stick skillet for about 10 minutes. Stir half of the Cajun spice into mayo in a small bowl and add as much salt and pepper as you'd like. Drizzle both sides of salmon with olive oil, sprinkle with rest of Cajun spice, and place on skillet for 2 minutes each side. Cut the bread and put on the mayo mix. Then put the salmon on the bread with tomato and cabbage.

13). Protein Pancakes

Ingredients:
1 cup Kodiak Power Pancakes
½ cup water
¼ cup maple syrup

Nutrition Facts:
Protein: 28g
Carbs: 115g
Fat: 4g
Total Calories: 518

How to Make It:
Mix the water and pancake mix in a bowl. Then put it on a hot skillet. Add syrup and whipped cream (optional)

14). Broiled Seasoned Salmon

Ingredients:
6 ounces of salmon fillet
Tiny bit of oregano and pepper
1 tbsp lemon juice
1 cup brown rice
2 cups raw spinach
½ cup diced tomato
2 tbsp balsamic vinaigrette

Nutrition Facts:
Protein: 45g
Carbs: 52g
Fat: 39g
Total Calories: 743

How to Make It:
Season the salmon with oregano and pepper, pour the lemon juice, and put it in the broiler for 5 minutes (you'll know it's done with the fish separates with a fork) Cook the rice according to the instructions (buy microwavable rice packs)

Place spinach and diced tomatoes on a plate and add balsamic vinaigrette and serve with the fish.

15). Awesome Salmon Salad

Ingredients
1 cups cooked, flaked salmon
2 hard-boiled eggs, crushed
1 red or green bell pepper, diced
1 cucumber, peeled, seeded, and diced
1/2 cup chopped onions
4 to 5 tablespoons mayonnaise, or enough to moisten
1/4 teaspoon cayenne pepper, optional
Salt and pepper
1/2 lemon, juiced

Nutrition Facts:
Protein: 42g
Carbs: 5g
Fat: 36g
Total Calories: 710g

How to Make It:
Toss the salmon and crushed hard boiled eggs. In another bowl mix the bell peppers, cucumbers, onion, and mayo and add the seasonings/spices and mix. Then add everything together in a salad bowl.

16). Chicken Burrito

Ingredients
1 skinless, boneless chicken breast
1 cup brown rice (microwavable)
½ cup asparagus
¼ cup diced tomato
¼ avocado
1 tbsp Swiss cheese
1 high fiber wrap

Nutrition Facts:
Protein: 37g
Carbs: 54g
Fat: 15g
Total Calories: 490

How to Make It:
Broil the chicken breast for 7 minutes and cook the rice according to the instructions. Steam the asparagus and dice the chicken, asparagus, tomato, and avocado. Put the rice, chicken, vegetables, and cheese on the wrap.

17). Mixed-Pepper & Chicken Pasta

Ingredients
1 skinless and boneless chicken breast
½ cup bow-tie pasta
1 teaspoon olive oil
1/8 cup green pepper
1/8 cup red pepper
1/8 cup yellow pepper
½ cup pasta sauce

Nutrition Facts:
Protein: 36g
Carbs: 54g
Fat: 11g
Total Calories: 456

How to Make It:
Broil chicken breast and dice it and cook the pasta according to the instructions. Heat a skillet on medium heat and add all of the peppers until they're tender and stir in the pasta sauce and let simmer for 5-10 minutes and serve over pasta.

18). Spicy Tilapia

Ingredients
½ teaspoon Chinese 5-spice powder
¼ pound tilapia fillets
¾ tbsp light brown sugar
3 teaspoons soy sauce
¼ tbsp. canola oil
1 scallion, sliced

Nutrition Facts:
Protein: 24g
Carbs: 17g
Fat: 6g
Total Calories: 175

How to Make It:
Sprinkle the spice powder on both sides of the tilapia fillets. Mix the brown sugar and soy sauce in a small bowl. Heat a skillet over medium heat and add the oil and then cook the tilapia for 2 minutes. Flip the tilapia and reduce the heat and add the soy and brown sugar mixture until it reaches a boil. Oncc it boils, remove it from the skillet and plate it and drizzle it with the sauce.

19). Greek Pita Pizza

Ingredients

6 ounces boneless, skinless chicken breast
1 pita bread
½ tbsp. olive oil
2 tbsp sliced olives
1 tsp red wine vinegar
½ clove garlic
¼ tsp oregano and basil
¼ cup spinach
2 tbsp feta cheese

Nutrition Facts:

Protein: 49g
Carbs: 15g
Fat: 36g
Total Calories:

How to Make It:

Broil the chicken breast. Then place it on the pita with all of the other ingredients and put in in the broiler for a few minutes (until the feta browns a little)

20). Muscle French Toast

Ingredients
4 slices bread
2 egg whites
2 whole eggs
1/3 cup fat free milk
2 scoops protein powder
½ teaspoon cinnamon
¼ cup maple syrup

Nutrition Facts:
Protein: 63g
Carbs: 89g
Fat: 11g
Total Calories: 703

How to Make It:
Mix the eggs, egg whites, protein powder, milk, and cinnamon. Then quickly put the bread in there and place it on a hot skillet until both sides are cooked.

Did You Find This Book Useful? Then Show Some Love!

I wanted to thank you for purchasing and reading this entire book. If you liked it, **please leave a 5-star rating** and feel free to email me at raza@thescienceofgettingripped.com if you have any questions.

Reviews are very important to us authors, and it only takes a minute to post. At the end of this book please post a review.

And don't forget to get your free bonus "The Dessert Report" when you visit my blog:

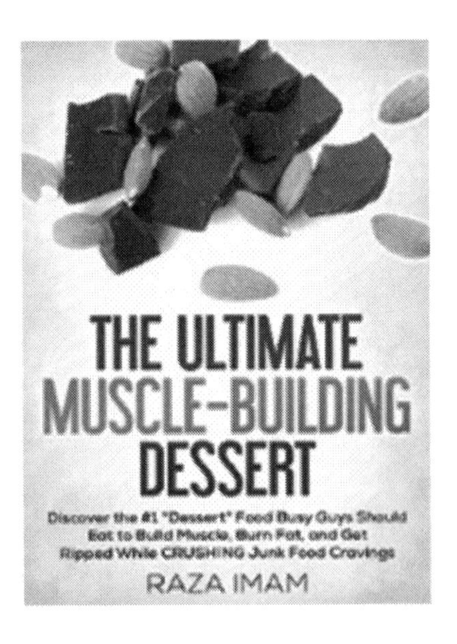

www.TheScienceofGettingRipped.com

Thank you in advance!

Made in the USA
Middletown, DE
07 December 2018